\'ker-,gi-ver\

(read in your voice)

Marti Steiner

For John...

Marti Steiner

\'ker-,giv-er\

Path to Resolution

Recovery

Path to Resolution

Blackdamp

Dad worked in the mines all his life, hot
in the Dark, sweating
inhaling Death.

He doesn't complain
about those who profited from that labor.
as he was dying.

No, his life was full
of Love.
His woman and those kids.
The redtick coons,
Ethereal hymn at church,
Moonlight on fresh fallen snow,
The red sun falling between the blue hills.

He doesn't complain to me,
Or to the nurses.
He just shifts in the bed,
adjusts his oxygen tube

and struggles to breath.
in the Dark, sweating
exhaling Life.

Marti Steiner

\'ker-,giv-er\

Respite

The boy and his mother showed up last Tuesday.
The woman elbowed her way in, gripping the casserole and
promptly put water on the stove for tea and asked where
the keys to the mower were.

That ruffled haired boy grinned as he quickly headed to the
barn.

I spent the morning picking up the place.
It was still messy,
a plethora of medicine bottle, bandages, and paperwork.
But I did get the dishes done.

The woman chatted about church gossip,
They ran out of communion last week, the knitting
missionaries think the pastor is dating a woman from a
church in the next county.

She pours a cup of Earl Grey, and opens the kitchen
curtains-
The blinding summer sun cutting the room like a carving
knife.

The mower hums, and she laughs
as she sweeps the floor and tells me
how one time her son locked the keys in the trunk while
they were camping, and
how nervous a coworker was
when he asked her on a date to the movies.

The steam from the cup of tea reflects white in the sun,
and I cannot help but laugh.
While my husband sleeps in the bedroom,
one foot firmly
in the grave.

Marti Steiner

\'ker-,giv-er\

The Gift

It's been two years since the diagnosis and today she forgot who I am.

Then, at 3:17 she looked up from the tv and called me by name,
and asked what was for dinner.
with smiling eyes, like she had just returned from a girls night out.

Before, we were angry, then depressed.
I didn't marry the person she was becoming.
She did not want me to become her caregiver-
she had always imagined us later, in our 80's,
wrinkled hands clasped on the front porch swing.

But these two years have also been a gift-
We focus on each day, what we have right now,
and are grateful.
We live life to the fullest, growing in each other.
And sometimes we forget.
I have lost myself to this woman,
And through this struggle
I see the profound blessing she is.

This morning, she sat up straight in the bed we've shared for 27 years,
Her hair reflecting gold and silver,

And she didn't recognize me.

To be fair, sometimes I don't recognize myself.

But, I've been preparing for this day. I thought I was ready.
Yet, I am broken inside.

Marti Steiner

Dependence

My younger brother and I knew
That it would be bad
When our mother brought home that case of Old Milwaukee.
Every other Friday.
No dinner tonight.

We knew to stay out of the way,
Unseen and silent
I would hold his hand under the pillow we shared.
And we dreamed of another space

Now our mother lies in her bed,
Yellow
Thin and bloated.
She has difficulty focusing.

As I check her bile tube,
Inspect for bruising,
And I have to wonder

How it came to be
That I am the one
Taking care of the mother
Who was no mother to me.

Marti Steiner

Cancer Sucks

Cancer Sucks.
Of course it fucking does!
Who designed that dumbass bumper sticker?
What idiot thinks we need to be reminded as
we cruise down the highway?
or sit in the hospital parking lot.

I sit, knuckles white on the steering wheel,
They match the snow on the manicured bushes.

Cancer will get my child.
That boy that formed inside me,
and smiled six weeks after his birth.

I know.
I know that cancer will take him.

All of that potential.
The talent.
His love.
Will soon be snuffed from this earth.

I have given the last 253 days everything...
the appointments,
the doctors,
the tests.
the chemicals pumped into my boy,
with knowing eyes.

Six weeks ago we asked him if he wanted to continue...
and he told us he was tired.
He would be better where he was going.

Marti Steiner

A gift, he made the choice
.

So we went to the beach, and laughed…
the warm sun smiling
as we gripped each other.
and would not let go.

Could I have been a better parent?
I cried, and cry.
my lungs are like carded wool,
i'm empty, barely going through the motions.
I am pissed at God.
Is this punishment to atone for my sins?
Fuck Him! Those are my sins alone, not this boys.

Perhaps those that suffer the most are those that are left.

Marti Steiner

Chromosome 21

We knew she was special
from the moment she was born.
Dark, curly hair,
eyes the color of the sky

Her soul is one of joy,
as this is what you first notice
and no one departs her presence without
becoming a better person.

I can't say it's been a basket of roses,
The countless doctor appointments,
The hospital stays,
The sideways stares.

Our routine is important
and it can be a terrible thing
if we stray, another difficult day.
Still a gift.

We've accounted for when we die,
but I dread the fact that we most likely
will outlive her.
What will I do then? Who will I be?

Marti Steiner

FUBAR

Years ago, I worried that he would buy the farm KIA.
But he's been a straight arrow,
forty-five years with me.

Now, we've had our share of hard times,
don't get me wrong-
but we've always been a team,
and with him and God's grace
we always worked through that stuff.

We prayed a lot.

He's had the cough for six months, and now
the VA tells us it's most likely Agent Orange.

That he's ate up.

Two months ago, they said there was a procedure,
but he keeps getting rescheduled.

I've read his lab report, his doctor's notes.
So much paperwork
I don't understand.

I called at 9am one morning six weeks ago,
To tell them he couldn't manage the pain anymore.
A nurse called back at 3:45-
His pills were in the mail, and he should receive them within
Five days.
What the shit?

The next day I called Hospice.
We still haven't seen a specialist

Marti Steiner

No hero's welcome when he came back from Nam,
and still a casualty of war.

This most honorable man,
my Love and Soulmate,
lies in this hospice bed,
with no regrets.
and smiles at me,
right now in this moment.

Forever

Marti Steiner

\'ker-,giv-er\

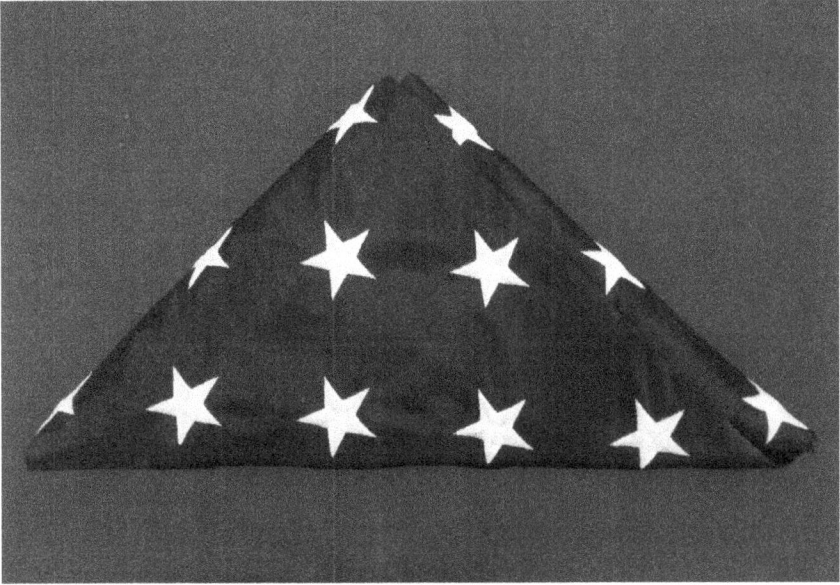

Marti Steiner

Falling

They call my seventeen year old daughter a junkie,
and that she deserves to die.
This gentle flax haired girl,
caught in a web of medical lies.

First, relief from a shattered leg she broke
while trying to save a tiny orange tabby kitten
stuck in a tree.

That oxycodone—Death's icy fingers-
numbed her nerves, yet she needed more.
She begged her doctors,
the rod and screws, her incision not yet healed.
She stole pills from her grandmother,
so she could sleep.

Then she shot up with a classmate.

When I found out, she told me she wasn't a
'bad addict,' and she had it under control.
She just needed it to function.

Where did we go wrong? How could this happen
to us?
I had no clue what to do, how to help her.

Then, five weeks ago she overdosed.
She was actively dying on the McDonald's bathroom floor,
next to a silver spoon and needle.

The paramedics saved her, and we immediately sent
her to rehab.
Where we found she was HIV +

Marti Steiner

\'ker-,giv-er\

Five months ago, my sweet girl was in the high school
marching band, sang in the church choir, and fell...
Saving a kitten.
She fell straight to Hell,
and that is where we are.

Dear God,

Please give this child the power to beat this, to fight the
very Devil himself. Give me the strength and knowledge
to help her. Let the church ladies whisper- I don't care.

Just save her. Save us.

Amen

Marti Steiner

\'ker-,giv-er\

Choose

We are damned.
My husband says,
we must pursue the third round.

But our daughter is tired.
Tired of the chemo.
Tired of this hospital.
Tired of this life.

Yet...
What if this is the round
that works?
What if she makes it through, and grows
Her hair?
Her color?
Her smile?

She will suffer the side effects no matter.
We will suffer the side effects no matter.

I am a hooded figure
holding the scythe for her child.

Marti Steiner

\'ker-,giv-er\

Circle

the doctors called.
they say when they pull
the ventilator,
She will pass.

but this is the fifth time,
and I have doubts
as I buy my one way five hour ticket
and prepare to stay at least a month.

She is stuborn, a good trait sometimes
She once told me She wanted
to live forever
and perhaps She will.
I love my Mother.

when I leave again
She will stop taking the meds
that keep her ticking
and again we will work with
in home Hospice
whom she will fire after I leave
and tell the docs
We are only after her money.

Marti Steiner

Last Man Standing

Mr Mason has been with us for two months. The state
admitted him after he caught his kitchen on fire...
A forgotten fried egg led to complete loss of freedom.

The day he arrived, I asked him if there was family,
Or perhaps a friend he'd like us to call.
He turned towards the open window,
And said,
"It's a terrible thing, you know.
To die alone. They're all gone.
I am the last man standing."

About a week into his stay,
Mr Mason gave up.

Well now, this won't do.
I told him that,
that he was brought to this place,
To be a friend I needed. Which is true.

They don't teach us that in training.

This happens far more often than people think.
In this age of digital interconnectedness,
and narcissistic social outpouring,
how many people are we truly bonded to?

The other aids trade residents with me.
They trade these lonely people, saying
they can't handle it.
Funny, because I see each one truly as a gift.

Marti Steiner

I sing when I wash their hair,
and bring them cards my kids make.
I ask them about their favorite food,
that favorite vacation,
their first kiss.
I genuinely want to learn.

Every person is a thread in the quilt of life,
each of us unique and connected,
every scrap needed for the masterpiece.
For there truly are no throwaway people,
Each has their story,
and I am ever grateful I will
hold Mr Mason's hand for
His last chapter.

Marti Steiner

\'ker-,giv-er\

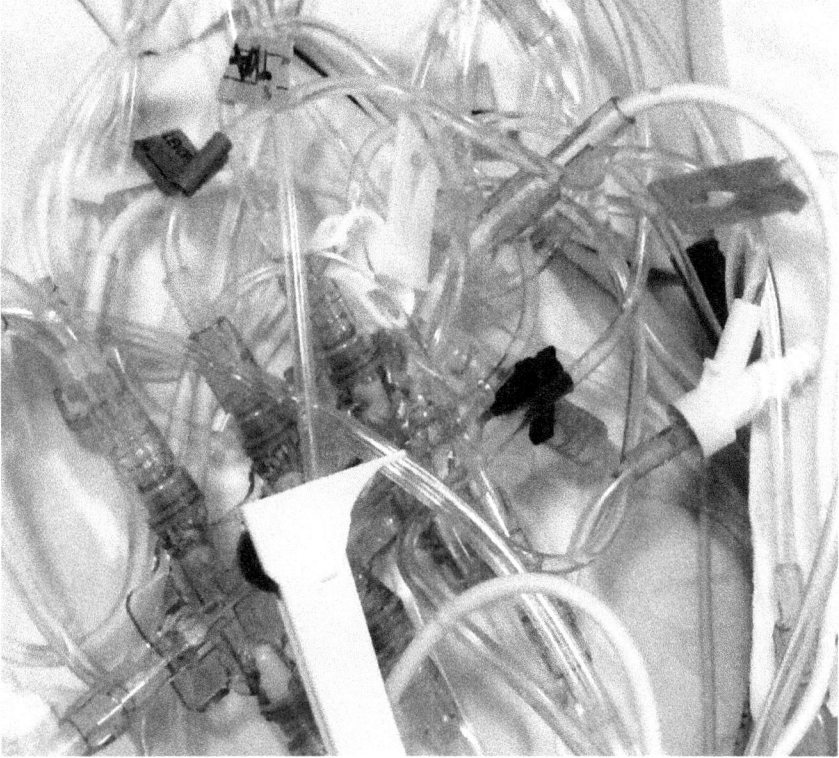

Marti Steiner

The Last Day

I've been staying with her the past three weeks.
Our baby was born dead, a complete knot in the cord.
Funny, because now I know I will never tie the knot
with her mamma.
I think she's crazy as shit...
Cries way too much.

I can't describe how I felt,
Because that little girl looked perfect.
Her fingers, and nose.
Her wispy hair.
Sleeping.
A part of me, that won't continue.

I've tried to help her mamma the best I can,
helped carry stuff, and
ordered takeout.
But she is way too needy, and
I can't deal with this shit.
Her stitches are almost healed,
and her own mamma will be coming tomorrow.

Everyone looks past me and tells her how
sorry they are she lost the baby.
What about how I am feeling?
No one gives a damn.
I'm outta here.

Marti Steiner

\'ker-,giv-er\

Recovery

Marti Steiner

Cath

I wait in this room,
as my man is prepped
to have dye wind
through the maze
of his arteries.

To his heart. Which
has worked to the point
of exhaustion.

He is tired.

Something isn't right,
I know this.

Marti Steiner

Beneficiary

Is he prepared?
The living will and will
What does he want?
Pondering his own mortality,
also has me thinking.

So listen my children
and promise me!
Turn me to dust-
No funeral,
No casket,
No service.

Only a potluck
attended by those
whom I've touched-
music and merriment,
for I will still be with you.

And read the following:

The Five Rules-
Love
Listen
Work
Share
Teach

Of these, love is the most difficult,
invest the bulk of your time on this.

Marti Steiner

Production Line

The patients are all branded
orange bracelets, personal info
and a UPC

Walked, then wheeled
following the corridor
of shop lights.
Scanned again and again.

I follow,
a disjointed symbiotic association
holding the forms
and asking questions.

Marti Steiner

Waiting Room

My love has been wheeled back.
Back to where they will crack his ribs,
Deflate his lungs,
Cool him, till he is dead.
A temporary death.
His brain forced to sleep.

At 6:12 in the cardiac waiting room,
The woman calls.
Calls to her husband, their children.

He's gone!
She cries out frantically,
Her daughter jolts to a stand.
What? What!
HE'S GONE.

They gasp, and pitch forward, as a unit.
Into the secured door, and down the hallway.
Blanched.
Eyes wide, awaiting death.

I am left in solitude.
Their baby's car seat still rocks,
Someone's forgotten phone vibrates
Again, and again.

Marti Steiner

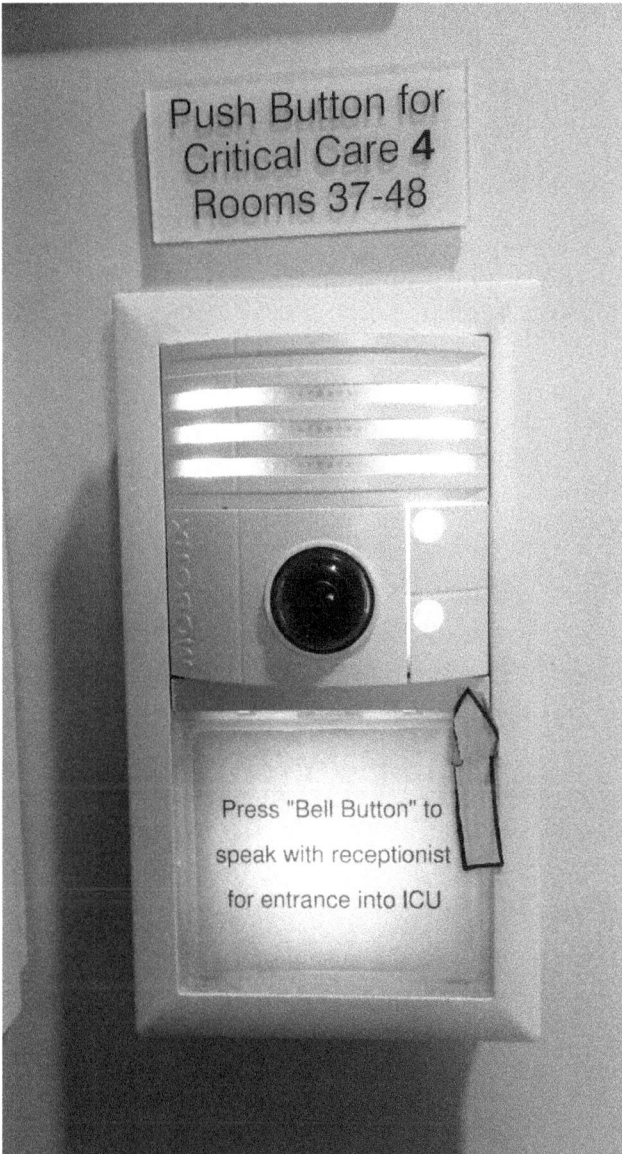

Marti Steiner

Procedure

I sit here and think.
You can not die.
I do not care what side affects you might have,
if they are temporary, or permanent.
You absolutely must not die.

It is a completely selfish demand,
for I am not done with you.

My soul tells me you will recover,
And be renewed, a chance to be reborn.
But my brain hears what the Doctors are saying,
that without this procedure lies
Certain death.

For death stalks us, like a cat
shifting its weight for a better view
before it attacks.

Marti Steiner

Lonely

We sit with tight faces,
waiting.
Our brains firing away
trying to keep the doubt silent.

One by one, we are called
back to our love, our friend
anxious, yet grateful
where we all begin our
recovery to a new life.

But I have to wonder
about those under the knife
who have
no one
waiting
in this too quiet, too bright room.

Marti Steiner

In Praise of Nurses

I sit in this waiting room, stressed.
I fret, and worry,
but mostly pray.

I beseech and bargain,
Please God
name your price,
heal this man.

Yet, what of those under the knife with
no one in this bright and tense room.

When the respirator is pulled, and they and focus
Who is there?
What do those who have had their insides rearranged
by a skilled surgeon think
when there is no lover, or friend
to rub their head,
hold their hand,
or simply sit and watch—
Praising God with each breath.

I surmise it is the overwhelmed nurse,
who understands healing is holistic.
Perhaps the nurse ultimately saves as many
as those with medical degrees.
Showing those that a human cares,
and giving hope.

Marti Steiner

Gossip

I find it very interesting,
how interesting people find us.
It is always a priority to keep us private,
shielded from this world,
For the other part of the public
has fangs,
and will even tear at the kids.

For a while, we were able to exist in peace,
our hearts mending in the quiet.
Yet, your heart needed more intervention-
The procedures,
The specialists,
The scalpel.

Your spark plugs needed rewired.

"Who will take care of you?" they asked.
And asked.
And asked.

And when you divulged, they knew,
a raised eyebrow, the knowing.
Honestly, a relief for the vast majority-
those who really care.
But a smug smile for a few.

No matter,
my own heart is full.
Lying beside you in this hospital bed,
As the morphine drips.

Marti Steiner

\'ker-,giv-er\

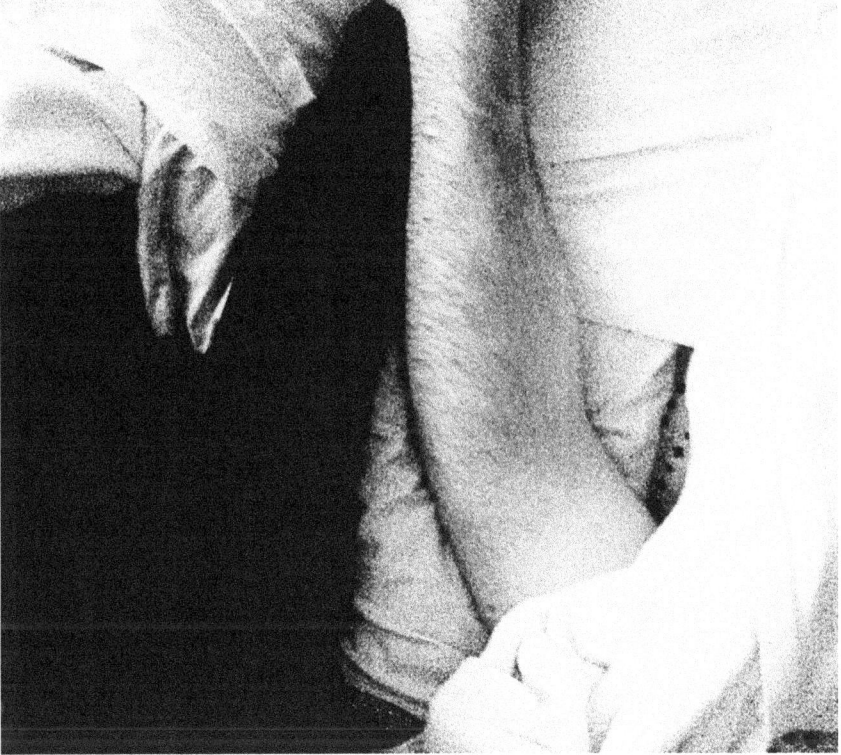

Marti Steiner

Ass out of U and Me

I am not his wife.
I am not his wife.
I am not his wife.
I am not his wife.
I am not his wife.
I am not his wife.
I am not his wife.
I am not his wife.
I am not his wife.
I am not his wife.
I am not his wife.
I am not his wife.
I am not his wife.
I am not his wife.
I am not his wife.
I am not his wife.
I am not his wife.
I am not his wife.
I am not his wife.
I am not his wife.
I am not his wife.
I am not his wife.
I am not his wife.
I am not his wife.
I am not his wife.
I am not his wife.

All in six days.

He's not interested,
so how fucking annoying is that?

Marti Steiner

In Praise of Snails

I see you are exhausted,
working
weights, the recumbent bike and treadmill
at a snail's pace.

Your blood sugar drops
so you sit and sweat
while eating an orange
looking disgruntled.

Yet inside, I am your cheerleader,
your Mascot.
Like a grinning parent,
bursting with pride and gratitude.

That this man is able to exceed
his goal of 2mph.
That he is dedicated to
completing the program.
That he is here
on this Earth at all.

All sing praise to those snails!

Marti Steiner

Life Change

Well now,
he's been rewired, so how
do we keep that muscle pumping?

new food, new workout, new meds. Check.
He's on it.

Less stress? This one will be the problem.
I cannot see him changing what he does.
He is driven to continually improve..
Himself,
His family,
His community.

I add to his stress, I know.
and I continually try to improve the way
I communicate,
but I will not walk on eggshells,
or pussyfoot about.

We are in a continued state of flux,
My focus is on regained health.
and sometimes I get incredibly frustrated,
as I see he does.

For it will take a long time

We have to look at both the narrow
and wide path to recovery…
What is here before us
and the future path.

Marti Steiner

Songs of the Era

heartbreak hotel,
can't you hear my heartbeat,
my heart has a mind of its own

walk this crowd
down memory lane,
their hearts pumping
on the recumbent bike,
free weights,
the treadmill
dreaming of a past life

as the baby, your soundtrack
would be different

open your heart,
where do broken hearts go
total eclipse of the heart.
the same songs, really
just 20 years apart

yet, you be-bop
with the rest.
muscle flexing,
blood forced within

Marti Steiner

\'ker-,giv-er\

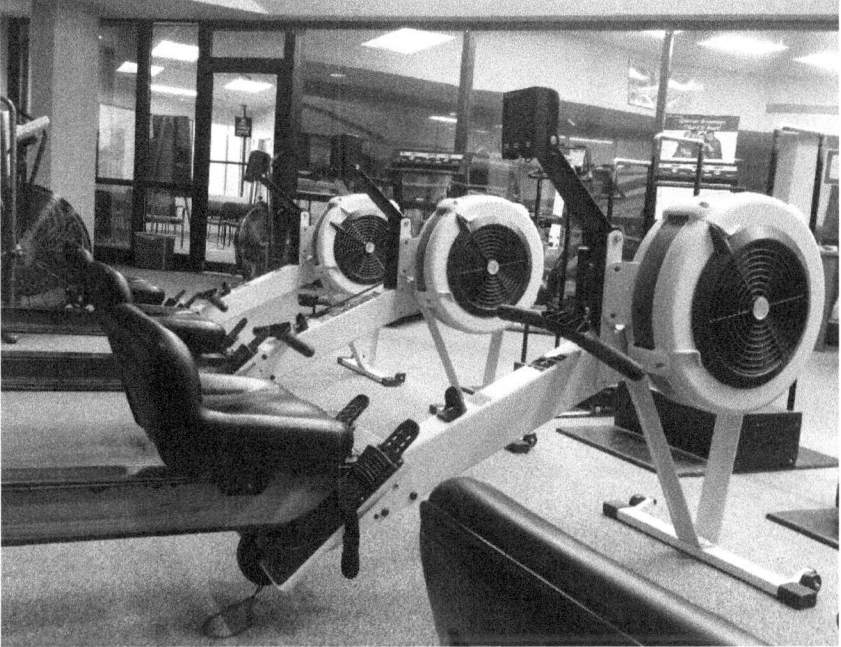

Marti Steiner

Free Will
or
48 Seconds
or
Put the Damn Cookie Down

The problem is me.

Mid-cookie, I frantically wonder if consuming that
homemade chocolate chip delight
made by that special friend
just for you

will actually reduce the time
I get to share with you here on this Earth.

I envision your life clock's time
Reduced.
The second hand skipping 48 seconds.
and I mentally scream in protest,
DON'T DO IT! PUT THE DAMN COOKIE DOWN!

There is no vocal exchange,
but my face must reflect what I am thinking,
because you hand me the remaining half,
and sheepishly grin.
A boy, with his hand in the cookie jar.

I know relationships are supposed to feel like freedom.
but I can't shake this need to violently vanquish
food with refined sugar from your grasp.

Truly, the problem lies not in your
ability to process insulin,

Marti Steiner

but my inability to cope
losing you those 48 seconds.

Marti Steiner

\'ker-,giv-er\

Dislike

I do not like being a caregiver.
The problem lies in the fact
that caregivers love.

We love these people,
to the point we
stop nurturing ourselves.
we second guess what we do,
and forget who we were.

Sometimes that former us is lost.

If we are very lucky,
our patient recovers
in all their Glory,
knowing they were well loved
and cared for.

But what of those of us
who Know
the recovery will be one
involving eternity?

Who will be their own caregiver
as they heal?

My heart cries for these.

Marti Steiner

A Change in Venue

Not as modern, that is evident.
The digital, virtual
Doesn't exist.

However,
Human interaction and personal education prevails.
Not the electric readout.
Devoid of the latest technology,
But perhaps the best for healing.

Marti Steiner

\ˈker-ˌgiv-er\

Just a

What box shall be checked?
What relationship am I?
Check the box 'Friend'.

I am the 'Friend'
then the side glance
(for 'Friend' = courtesan)
Nevermind I am named in his living will.

Once again I am
forgotten in the waiting room.

Marti Steiner

Beard

Those six days in the hospital
Were the longest you had ever
Gone without shaving.

An interesting fact,
Considering you've been a man for so long.

Now you wonder,
Do you like it?

You hate the grey, but
I see each silver glint
as a gift.
As a chance to grow wise,
to have the opportunity to learn.

You say you hate the way it
pricks your face,
how it scratches.

You look in the mirror,
and think about your work ahead.
Ponder aloud if it will affect the way people
think about you.

Do you like it?
You don't know.

But you haven't shaved.

Marti Steiner

\'ker-,giv-er\

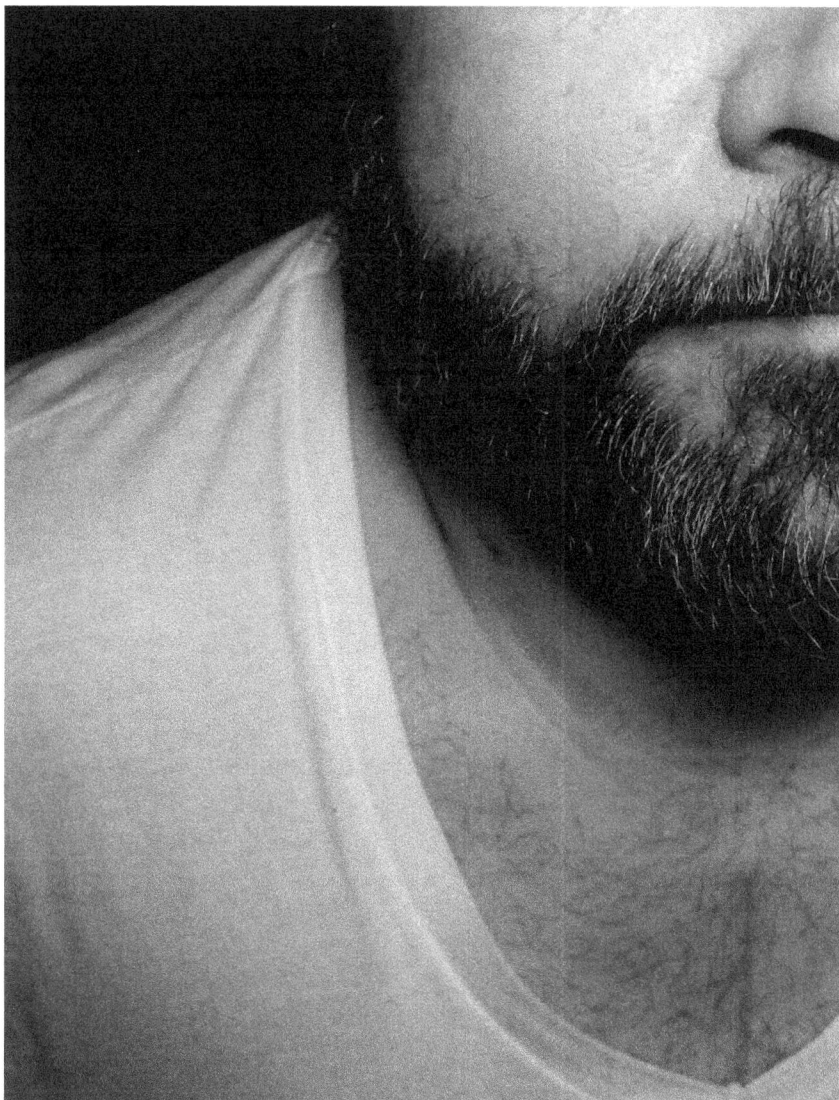

Marti Steiner

Gratitude

I cannot describe
my gratitude you choose
to change.

It isn't easy,
for we have lived our life
in denial.

So many do not
decide to walk that path
with faith.

Emerging from the
baptismal font of life
born again.

Marti Steiner

The Passing of the Torch

The moment has come for me to
pass the torch to you.
You have been dedicated
to your training.
Eating right and sweating,
working to a new life.
You are ready to take full responsibility
for you.
The accolades all well-earned.

To not be needed is an adjustment though.

Marti Steiner

\'ker-,giv-er\

To all Caregivers...

Marti Steiner

Peace

Marti Steiner

\'ker-,giv-er\

A portion of the proceeds will be donated to provide free training for Recovery Coaching

Build your community.

Engage.

Marti Steiner

\'ker-,giv-er\

Thank You

Marti Steiner

\'ker-,giv-er\

For more information about the author-

Marti Steiner

m.facebook.com/JourneyIntoMyWorld

Marti Steiner

\'ker-,giv-er\

Marti Steiner

www.ingramcontent.com/pod-product-compliance
Lightning Source LLC
Chambersburg PA
CBHW060627210326
41520CB00010B/1507